Poisoning Treatment

How to Approach Poisoning Patients, Unknown Substance & Common Poisons and Their Management In Emergency

Dan Phillips PhD

~DEDICATION~

~LARRY~

For your unwavering support, encouragement, and friendship. Your presence in my life has been a constant source of inspiration. Thank you for your invaluable kindness and belief in my journey. This book is a token of appreciation for your enduring friendship and steadfast encouragement.

TABLE OF CONTENT

CHAPTER 1

Introduction to Poisoning Treatment:

Throughout human history, poisoning occurrences have posed a constant threat, frequently occurring suddenly and necessitating quick medical intervention. This thorough guide to poisoning treatment's first chapter delves into the critical area of poison management in emergency situations, emphasizing how critical it is to act quickly and decisively in order to lessen the potentially fatal effects of poison exposure.

Knowing How Serious Poisoning Events Are:

Accidental ingestion, inhalation, absorption, or injection of toxic substances—both naturally occurring and man-made—can cause poisoning episodes. These substances, which are also known as poisons, might include anything from poisonous plants and animal bites to everyday household chemicals and prescriptions. The possibility of severe injury or even death from poisoning, regardless of the source, emphasizes the importance of having a solid understanding of poison management, especially in emergency situations.

The Need for Prompt Intervention:

This guide's first chapter emphasizes how critical it is to act quickly in poisoning cases. In contrast to many medical emergencies, which may present with a slow onset of symptoms, poisoning can result in severe reactions that require quick attention. Treatment delays may worsen the poison's effects and increase the risk of death or irreparable damage. As a result, treating toxin exposure quickly and effectively is essential to preventing long-term health issues and saving lives.

Insufficient Information and the Requirement for Schooling:

The difficulties involved in treating poisoning occurrences may be made worse by the general public's and even healthcare professionals' ignorance of poison management. Delivering appropriate and effective treatment requires knowledge of the precise antidotes, decontamination protocols, and supportive care needed for various forms of poisoning. Because of this, the first chapter highlights how crucial it is for first responders, healthcare professionals, and even individuals to receive education and training so they can be prepared to act quickly and effectively in the event of a poisoning.

The Varying Character of Poisoning Agents:

The wide variety of chemicals that can cause toxicity is one of the most noticeable features of poisoning episodes. The potential origins of poisoning are almost endless, ranging from everyday household items like cosmetics and cleaning solutions to more unusual compounds like industrial chemicals and plant toxins.

This variability presents a serious obstacle to identifying the precise poison and providing the right therapy, as was covered in the first chapter. Hence, a basic prerequisite for handling poisoning situations successfully is a solid understanding of toxicology and toxin detection.

Poison Control Centers' Function:

The importance of poison control centers is also emphasized in the introduction to poisoning therapy. In cases of suspected poisoning, these specialist services are essential in giving prompt support and direction to medical professionals and the general population. Poison control centers play a major role in precise diagnosis and successful intervention because of their access to current knowledge on dangerous compounds, antidotes, and treatment regimens. The chapter emphasizes how crucial it is to work together with these centers in order to maximize patient outcomes and care.

Comprehensive Method for Treating Poisoning:

The first chapter emphasizes the use of an integrated approach to poisoning treatment. The complex nature of poison exposure means that multiple healthcare specialties, such as emergency medicine, toxicology, pharmacology, and critical care, frequently need to work together for optimal therapy. In order to guarantee a thorough and well-coordinated response to poisoning situations, the chapter emphasizes the necessity of clear communication and cooperation among various specialists.

Implications for Public Health:

The wider public health consequences of insufficient poison control are also included in the introduction to poisoning treatment. Incidents of poisoning can put a strain on healthcare systems and resources in addition to having an effect on specific patients and their families. The possibility of widespread poisonings, as observed in instances of water or food contamination, emphasizes the necessity of strong public health policies and emergency action plans to handle such situations.

Conclusion

To sum up, the first chapter of this guide emphasizes how critical poison management is in emergency situations. In order to minimize possible harm and preserve lives, poisoning occurrences require quick and effective actions. Important elements in this process are emphasized, including the need for prompt treatment, the variety of poisoning agents, and the function of poison control centers. The chapter acts as a call to action, stressing the importance of cooperation, education, and a thorough approach to poisoning treatment in order to guarantee the best possible results for people who have been exposed to harmful substances. Readers will delve deeper into the precise tactics and interventions that support efficient poison management in a variety of settings as the upcoming chapters are revealed.

CHAPTER 2

Initial Assessment and Triage of Poisoning Patients:

- Steps for a systematic approach to poisoned patients

- Rapid assessment techniques to identify critical cases

When faced with potentially poisoned patients, a systematic and rapid approach is critical to ensure the best possible outcomes. This chapter outlines the steps for a systematic approach to poisoned patients and provides rapid assessment techniques to identify critical cases.

2.1 Steps for a Systematic Approach to Poisoned Patients

1. Scene Safety:

- Ensure your safety and that of the patient and any bystanders. If the scene is unsafe, wait for assistance or until the environment is secure.

2. Primary Survey:

- Assess the patient's airway, breathing, and circulation (ABCs).

- Ensure an open airway. If the patient is unconscious, check for obstructions and provide basic life support if necessary.

- Evaluate breathing and administer oxygen if indicated.

- Check circulation, assessing the pulse and blood pressure. Look for signs of shock.

3. History:

- Gather information from the patient, bystanders, or medical records to understand the circumstances of poisoning.

- Identify the toxic substance, the amount ingested, the time of exposure, and the patient's medical history.

4. Physical Examination:

- Perform a thorough physical examination to identify signs and symptoms of poisoning, such as abnormal vital signs, altered mental status, or specific clinical findings related to the toxin.

5. Decontamination:

- Initiate decontamination procedures if necessary. This may involve removing contaminated clothing, flushing skin or eyes with water, or inducing vomiting as appropriate.

6. Stabilization:

- Provide supportive care to stabilize the patient's condition. This may include administering intravenous fluids, supplemental oxygen, or medications to control symptoms.

7. Laboratory and Diagnostic Tests:

- Order specific tests, such as blood tests, urine tests, or imaging, to identify the toxic substance, assess organ function, and guide treatment decisions.

2.2 Rapid Assessment Techniques to Identify Critical Cases

1. Glasgow Coma Scale (GCS):

- Use the GCS to assess the patient's level of consciousness. A lower GCS score may indicate severe poisoning.

2. Vital Signs:

- Monitor vital signs, including heart rate, respiratory rate, blood pressure, and oxygen saturation. Abnormal vital signs may signal critical cases.

3. Toxidromes:

- Recognize specific toxidromes, which are clusters of symptoms and signs associated with certain types of poisoning (e.g., anticholinergic,

cholinergic, sympathomimetic, opioid toxidromes). Identifying these can guide treatment.

4. Serum Toxin Levels:

- Measure serum levels of specific toxins when available. Elevated levels may confirm poisoning and help assess severity.

5. ECG (Electrocardiogram):

- Perform an ECG to detect cardiac abnormalities, especially in cases of drug or chemical exposures that affect the heart (e.g., sodium channel blockers or certain toxins).

A systematic approach to poisoned patients, combined with rapid assessment techniques, is crucial in identifying critical cases and providing appropriate care. This allows healthcare professionals to intervene effectively, administer antidotes, and manage the patient's condition, ultimately improving the chances of a successful outcome.

CHAPTER 3

Recognition and Management of Common Poisons:

- Detailed information on frequently encountered toxins

- Signs, symptoms, and appropriate interventions for each poison

When it comes to poison control, being able to quickly identify and handle frequently encountered poisons is critical. This thorough guide's third chapter is devoted to giving complete information on common poisons, explaining each one's symptoms, indicators, and suitable interventions. Through providing thorough knowledge to individuals, first responders, and healthcare professionals, this chapter seeks to enable prompt and accurate reactions to poisoning occurrences, ultimately improving patient outcomes.

Knowledge of Common Poisons:

We explore a variety of compounds that are frequently linked to poisoning episodes in this chapter. There are many different types of possible poisons, ranging from commonplace substances like medicines and cleaning supplies to naturally occurring toxins found in plants and animals. A thorough understanding of these poisons is necessary. This chapter provides readers with an understanding of the kinds of compounds that often result in poison exposure, which lays the groundwork for efficient poison management.

Symptoms and Signs: Indications for a Diagnosis:

The capacity to recognize the signs and symptoms that appear after exposure is essential for the identification and management of common poisons. An extensive examination of the different clinical manifestations connected to every kind of toxin is given in this chapter. The indicators that may indicate the presence of a particular poisonous substance—such as changes in vital signs, neurological symptoms, gastrointestinal distress, skin manifestations, and more—will be explained to readers. The chapter stresses that accurate diagnosis requires careful observation and comprehensive assessment.

Adapting Treatment to Toxins: Appropriate Interventions

There is no such thing as a one-size-fits-all strategy when it comes to toxin control. In order to successfully counteract the effects of certain poisons, different actions are required. Beyond just identifying symptoms, Chapter 3 provides thorough advice on the right course of action for every poison. Through the use of activated charcoal, gastric lavage, emesis induction, supportive care, and specific antidotes, readers will obtain a comprehensive understanding of the interventions that are most likely to result in favorable outcomes for patients exposed to common poisons.

Typical Poisons and How They're Managed:

1. Overdose on Acetaminophen (Paracetamol):

Abdominal pain, nausea, vomiting, disorientation, and jaundice are some of the signs and symptoms.

- Interventions: monitoring liver function, giving supportive care, and administering N-acetylcysteine.

2. Home Cleaners (Ammonia, Bleach, and Other Chemicals):

Coughing, eye and skin irritation, and respiratory distress are the signs and symptoms.

- Interventions: irrigation of the eyes, supportive respiratory care, and quick removal from exposure.

3. Pesticides using Organophosphates:

- Muscle twitching, salivation, lacrimation, urine, and feces are signs and symptoms.

Interventions: decontamination, respiratory assistance, and the administration of atropine and pralidoxime.

4. Industrial Accidents, Smoke Inhalation, Cyanide Exposure):

- Headache, dizziness, fast breathing, and cherry-red skin are some of the signs and symptoms.

- Interventions: Sodium thiosulfate, hydroxocobalamin, and supportive care.

5. Venomous snake bites, or envenomation:

- Pain, bruising, swelling, and changes in blood clotting are the signs and symptoms.

Interventions: Identifying the type of snake, administering a particular antivenom, and tending to wounds.

Education and Prevention: A Holistic Perspective:

In addition to providing readers with the information they need to handle common toxins, Chapter 3 highlights the need of education and prevention. People can limit the risk of exposure by taking proactive precautions and making educated decisions by being aware of the chemicals that often result in poisoning cases. In order to minimize poisoning-related emergencies, this chapter emphasizes the importance of public education campaigns, appropriate storage practices for potentially dangerous materials, and safety precautions.

Final Thought: Facilitating Efficient Poison Management:

To sum up, Chapter 3 is a vital tool for identifying and handling common toxins. This chapter gives people and healthcare practitioners the tools they need to react quickly and effectively to poisoning occurrences by going into great detail about commonly encountered poisons, their signs and symptoms, and suitable interventions. This chapter makes a substantial contribution to the overall objective of improving patient outcomes in poison exposure cases by placing a heavy emphasis on customized therapies, precise diagnoses, and prevention measures. Readers will be well-prepared to confidently and competently negotiate the challenges of poison control as they work their way through this book.

CHAPTER 4

Decontamination Techniques for
Poison Ingestion:

- Methods of gastrointestinal decontamination (activated charcoal, gastric lavage, etc.)

- Criteria for selecting decontamination methods based on poison type and timing

Decontamination is an important part of poisoning case management since it tries to eliminate or lessen the body's absorption of harmful substances. The kind of toxin consumed, when it was consumed, and the patient's clinical state are among the variables that determine which decontamination techniques are best. This chapter examines several gastrointestinal decontamination techniques and describes how to choose the best one for a certain circumstance.

Guaranteed Techniques for Digestive Decontamination

Interventions that stop ingested contaminants from being absorbed deeper into the gastrointestinal tract are known as gastrointestinal decontamination. The two most often employed techniques are gastric lavage and the introduction of activated charcoal.

I. Activated Charcoal:

An very powerful adsorbent that attaches itself to toxins in the digestive system and keeps them from entering the bloodstream is activated charcoal. It can be given orally or via a nasogastric tube. Then the feces get rid of the charcoal-toxin combination. Lots of medications, chemicals, and some poisons can be effectively adsorbed by activated charcoal.

2. Lavage of the stomach:

A tube is inserted into the stomach during gastric lavage, also referred to as stomach pumping, in order to eliminate food particles. Any leftover toxins are aspirated along with the fluids after the stomach is cleansed several times with either saline or water. The best results from gastric lavage occur soon after a potentially fatal dose of poison is consumed and when the toxin has not yet fully absorbed.

3.   Complete Irrigation of the Bowel:

During whole bowel irrigation, a polyethylene glycol solution is given to the patient in an effort to promote the fast passage of food through the digestive system. It is helpful for significant ingestions of iron or other toxic compounds, as well as for drugs with an enteric coating or prolonged release.

4. Induction of Ememesis:

The process of emesis induction entails giving drugs (such ipecac syrup) to induce vomiting. However, because of the possibility of problems, lack of effectiveness, and aspiration risk, this procedure is generally not advised.

5. Cathartic + Activated Charcoal:

Toxin removal can be improved by mixing activated charcoal with a cathartic, which is a drug that stimulates bowel motions. The cathartic expedites the toxins' transit through the intestines while the charcoal binds them.

Selection Criteria for Decontamination Techniques

A thorough assessment of a number of variables, such as the type of poison, the date of consumption, the patient's clinical state, and any contraindications, is necessary before selecting the best decontamination technique.

1. Type of Poison:

The affinities of various poisons for adsorption onto activated charcoal differ. Charcoal-binding substances, like some medications, can be efficiently eliminated. On the other hand, materials like heavy metals that don't bind to charcoal react less well to this technique.

2. Ingestion Timing:

Decontamination methods become less efficient with the passage of time following poison consumption. While gastric lavage is generally helpful in the first few hours after ingestion, activated charcoal is most effective in the first hour following ingestion. Postponed presentations could make these techniques less useful or possibly harmful.

3. Patient's Clinical Condition: It is important to take into account the patient's general health, including their degree of consciousness, airway status, and aspiration risk. It is not recommended to perform gastric lavage or induce emesis in a patient who is unconscious or at risk of aspirating.

4. Risks and Contraindications:

Certain medical disorders and situations may make decontamination procedures contraindicated or raise their dangers. For example, if caustic substances are consumed, gastric lavage might not be the best course of action because it could worsen tissue damage.

5. Considerations Particular to Substances:

Selecting the appropriate decontamination techniques can be aided by knowledge of the properties of the particular poison, its rate of absorption, and its countermeasures.

For example, if the drug has a low toxicity profile or a specialized antidote is available, decontamination might not be required.

6. Patient collaboration: Patient cooperation is necessary for the administration of activated charcoal and the induction of emesis. Occasionally, patients might not be willing or able to comply, which makes these techniques useless.

In conclusion, choosing the right decontamination technique is an important choice to make while handling poisoning cases. To choose the best course of action, healthcare professionals must carefully consider a number of aspects, including the type of poison, when the ingestion occurred, the patient's clinical status, and any potential contraindications. When applied correctly, intestinal cleansing techniques such as gastric lavage and the administration of activated charcoal can dramatically lower the absorption of toxins. To guarantee the best possible patient care, these techniques should only be used sparingly and after carefully weighing the risks and advantages of each.

CHAPTER 5

Enhanced Elimination Strategies:

- Focus on enhancing toxin elimination (hemodialysis, urinary alkalinization, etc.)

- Indications, contraindications, and protocols for enhanced elimination techniques

When exposed to some toxic substances or experiencing acute

poisoning, normal supportive care and antidotal treatments might not be enough to stop serious harm or even death. This thorough guide's fifth chapter explores improved elimination procedures, providing a targeted look at methods intended to hasten the body's excretion of toxins. This chapter provides healthcare practitioners with a comprehensive grasp of when and how to use these advanced therapies to enhance patient outcomes, with a focus on indications, contraindications, and specific procedures.

A Range of Improved Elimination Methods:

The application of improved elimination techniques is a significant development in the field of poison control. These methods take advantage of the body's normal filtration, excretion, and elimination mechanisms to help hasten the removal of pollutants. Although the precise techniques differ, they all aim to reduce the possibility of prolonged exposure and the harm that certain toxic compounds may cause as a result.

Determination and Indications:

The first section of Chapter 5 explores the signs that should make improved elimination tactics a priority. These methods might be crucial in situations where a substance's toxicity is extremely high or when the pace of removal through normal metabolic processes is sluggish. The chapter describes conditions where improved elimination may be crucial, including drug overdoses, exposure to drugs with extended half-lives, or circumstances where normal remedies are not adequate to avert serious injury.

Restriction and Safety Procedures:

Even though improved elimination techniques can be effective instruments, there are risks involved. The contraindications that need to be carefully considered before putting these strategies into practice are thoroughly examined in this chapter. To guarantee the safety and suitability of improved elimination therapies, factors like underlying medical disorders, impaired organ function, and possible drug interactions need to be assessed.

Hemodialysis: Cleaning the Blood of Toxins:

Hemodialysis is one of the main improved elimination methods discussed in this chapter. Through a sophisticated filtering process, toxins are removed directly from the bloodstream during this operation. The chapter offers a thorough examination of the conditions that warrant hemodialysis, the kinds of toxins that can be successfully removed, and the detailed instructions needed to carry out the process. The chapter also discusses the potential risks of hemodialysis and the significance of appropriate vascular access.

Renal Excretion Enhanced by Urinary Alkalinization:

In this chapter, another important procedure that is highlighted is urinary alkalinization. By changing the urine's pH, this tactic can increase the excretion of some harmful compounds. The mechanics underlying urine alkalinization, the particular applications for which it is indicated, and the procedures for reaching and preserving the appropriate urinary pH are all explained in this chapter. To give a thorough knowledge, possible hazards and limitations of this procedure are also covered.

Additional Enhanced Elimination Methods:

Other important improved elimination procedures, including multiple-dose activated charcoal, forced diuresis, and extracorporeal approaches, are covered in this chapter. The indications, contraindications, and procedural protocols are applied to each technique. Through the chapter's thorough explanation of these tactics, medical practitioners are better equipped to decide which ones to apply in various poisoning situations.

Result: A Diverse Method for Handling Poison:

The demand to acknowledge improved elimination mechanisms as essential elements of a comprehensive strategy to poison management is made in the concluding chapter of Chapter 5. Even though these methods are cutting edge, when used carefully and intelligently, they can have a major positive effect on patient outcomes in situations where toxicity is severe. The intricate interactions between indications, contraindications, and procedural details allow medical professionals to use enhanced elimination strategies as effective weapons in their toolbox to combat poisoning occurrences. Readers will gain the information and skills necessary to confidently and precisely negotiate the challenges of toxin elimination as they work through this book.

CHAPTER 6

Supportive Care and Symptomatic Treatment:

- **Importance of managing symptoms and complications in poisoning cases**

- **Strategies for maintaining vital functions and addressing organ system involvement**

Effective supportive care and symptomatic therapy are just as important in handling poisoning cases as certain antidotes and cleaning methods. A variety of symptoms and consequences may arise from poisoning occurrences, necessitating close observation and prompt medical attention. This chapter describes methods for preserving vital functions and addressing organ system involvement, as well as how critical it is to manage symptoms and complications in poisoning instances.

Importance of Symptom and Complication Management

Cases of poisoning can take many different forms, impacting different organ systems and producing a wide range of symptoms. It is imperative to promptly and appropriately handle these symptoms for multiple reasons:

1. Avoiding More Damage:
If these toxins are not handled, they can gradually harm tissues or organs. Controlling symptoms can lessen long-term effects and stop these harms from getting worse.

2. Comforting the Affected Area:
feelings of poisoning can include pain, discomfort, and unsettling feelings. The comfort and general

well-being of the patient are enhanced by effective symptom management.

3.   Stabilizing   the   Patient: Symptomatic treatment aids in keeping the patient stable and stops potentially fatal complications from arising.

4. Assisting in the Diagnosis:
Important hints on the underlying toxin can be found in the severity and type of symptoms, which can help with precise diagnosis and focused treatment.

5. Supporting the Body's Natural Defenses: By strengthening the body's

defenses against detoxification and recuperation, supportive care techniques can improve the prognosis for their patients.

Methods for Preserving Essential Activities and Handling Organ System Involvement

1. Control of Airways:

Preserving a patent and unobstructed airway is crucial. Intubation and mechanical ventilation may be necessary for patients who are unconscious or exhibiting altered mental status in order to guarantee proper oxygenation and ventilation.

Tip 2. Heart Support:

Certain poisons may result in hypotension, arrhythmias, or other problems with the heart. Vasopressors, intravenous fluids, and other drugs could be required to keep the heart rate and blood pressure stable.

3. Observation of the Nerve System:

Neurological symptoms that include paralysis, altered awareness, or seizures need to be closely watched and treated as necessary. It might be necessary to take sedatives, anticonvulsants, and other drugs.

4. Help for the Digestive System:

Diarrhea, vomiting, and other digestive problems can cause electrolyte imbalances and dehydration. It can be necessary to replenish fluids and electrolytes in order to preserve equilibrium.

5. Support for Renal Function:

It is possible for toxins to affect renal function and cause acute kidney damage. Renal problems can be identified and treated with the aid of urine output, electrolyte monitoring, and renal function tests.

6. Support for Hepatic Function:

A prevalent condition in many poisoning instances is liver damage. In supportive care, the liver is protected and supported through therapies and ongoing monitoring of liver function tests.

7. Control of Metabolism and Acid-Base

The body's acid-base equilibrium and metabolism can be upset by toxins. It is essential to treat these imbalances with the right drugs and therapies.

8. Control of Temperature:

There are certain poisons that might cause hypo- or hyperthermia. Cooling or heating techniques are examples of temperature regulation tactics that aid in preserving a normal body temperature.

9. Handling Pain:

Pain and suffering are frequent side effects of poisoning. The comfort and general well-being of the patient are enhanced by effective pain management.

10. Assistance with Psychology:

Patients and their family may experience psychological discomfort as a result of poisoning episodes. To handle these care-related issues, psychotherapy and emotional support are crucial.

Results

Coordinating symptomatic treatment with supportive care is essential for successfully managing poisoning situations. In addition to lowering the chance of long-term harm, healthcare professionals can enhance patient outcomes by treating symptoms, avoiding complications, and preserving essential functions. A thorough understanding of toxicology and medical treatment, along with a customized approach to each patient's condition, guarantee that the patient receives the best care possible during a trying and crucial time.

CHAPTER 7

Toxicological Antidotes and

Specific Therapies:

- In-depth discussion of antidotes and specific treatments for certain toxins

- Dosages, administration routes, and precautions for antidote use

The science and art of poison control are always changing because of new discoveries in toxicology that result in tailored treatments and specialized antidotes that can quickly reverse the effects of toxic substances. This thorough guide's seventh chapter dives deeply into the topic of toxicological countermeasures and particular treatments, providing a detailed analysis that examines the nuances of these measures. This chapter provides healthcare workers with the necessary information and skills to effectively use antidotes and particular treatments, thereby saving lives and minimizing the consequences of poisoning episodes. These include exact dosages and administration methods as well as important precautions.

Remedies: A Range of Deliverance:

In the event of severe poisoning, antidotes provide a glimmer of hope by acting to neutralize or counteract the effects of particular poisons. This chapter presents a wide range of countermeasures, each carefully designed to counteract the deleterious effects of certain poisons. Through an analysis of the mechanisms of action and an emphasis on their critical function, the chapter opens up a more thorough comprehension of how antidotes can be used to lessen the severe effects of poisoning.

In-depth Doses and Administration Pathways: Accuracy in Action:

When administering antidotes and targeted medicines, accuracy is crucial. This chapter covers every detail, giving readers exact dosages for different age groups and ways of administration (oral, intravenous, intramuscular, and so on). Healthcare practitioners may make sure that the antidotes are administered successfully and efficiently and maximize their ability to counteract the toxic effects by following these dosages and routes.

Warnings, Precautions, and Possible Difficulties: Guaranteeing Safety:

The chapter recognizes how crucial it is to provide antidotes safely and cautiously. There are potential problems, precautions, and warnings specific to each antidote. This chapter guides readers through the complexities of using antidotes, emphasizing particular contraindications, possible side effects, and important safety measures. Healthcare providers can reduce the possibility of unintentional negative effects and give antidotes with confidence by being aware of and adept at navigating these subtleties.

Instances of Countermeasures and Particular Treatments:

1. An Overdose of Opioids with Naloxone:

- Intranasal or intramuscular injection as the dosage and mode of administration.

- Cautions and Safety Measures: Risk of titrating in cases of severe overdose, in addition to withdrawal symptoms.

2. Flumazenil for Overdosage of Benzodiazepines:

IV injection is the method of administration and dosage.

- Cautions & Precautions: Patients with a history of epilepsy may experience seizures.

3. Antibodies specific to Digoxin for Toxicity: - Acute intravenous infusion is the recommended dosage and mode of administration.

- Cautions & Precautions: During administration, keep an eye out for hypersensitivity responses.

The recommended dosage and method of administration for Prussian Blue in cases of radioactive cesium or thollium ingestion is oral administration.

- Warnings and Precautions: Keep an eye out for any adverse gastrointestinal symptoms.

Final Thought: Directing Accuracy for Ideal Results:

To sum up, Chapter 7 is a knowledge guiding light for medical practitioners navigating the complicated world of toxicological counter-adjustments and targeted treatments. Through an exploration of the mechanisms underlying antidotal activities, dosages, methods of administration, and crucial precautions, this chapter equips readers to utilize these therapies with accuracy and assurance. The chapter's thorough insights empower medical practitioners to maximize the efficacy of antidotes and targeted medicines, which are constantly pushing the frontiers of poison control. By adding these cutting-edge therapies to their toolkit, professionals can have a significant influence on patient outcomes, changing the game against

harmful chemicals and offering hope
in the field of poison management.

CHAPTER 8

Handling New and Emerging Toxins and Unknown Substances

For healthcare professionals, encounters with unknown drugs and new poisons pose special problems. In these cases, a careful yet informed approach together with quick and methodical examination are crucial. This chapter describes how to identify unknown drugs, how to treat patients initially, and how to deal with the problems that arise from unexpected or novel harmful exposures.

Means of Determining Unknown Substances and Offering Preliminary Care

When handling an unknown chemical, a methodical strategy is needed that emphasizes information collecting, safeguarding medical professionals, and starting supportive care:

1. Scene Safety and Protection: Make sure that medical staff is wearing the proper personal protective equipment (PPE) before interacting with a patient

who has been exposed to an unknown material.

2. Evaluation of the Patient:
Assess the patient's vital signs first, then deal with any imminent hazards to their life. Make a note of any outward indications or symptoms that could provide you information about the chemical in question.

3. Collect Information: If at all possible, conduct an interview with the patient to learn more about the circumstances surrounding the exposure. Inquire about the exposure's cause, path, duration, and any symptoms you may have had.

4. Consult Resources: Based on the patient's presentation and medical history, identify possible chemicals and their effects by using readily available resources, such as toxicology databases, medical literature, or poison control centers.

5. Physical Examination: Perform a comprehensive physical examination to find any particular clinical indications or symptoms linked to recognized poisons.

6. Preliminary Care:
To stabilize the patient's state, start with symptomatic treatment and

supportive care. Prioritize preserving essential bodily processes, controlling symptoms, and dealing with issues as they appear.

7. Sample Collection: If practical and safe, gather samples of the unidentified material for additional examination and identification. Experts can identify the harmful agent and its characteristics with the use of these samples.

8. Monitor and Adjust: Constantly keep an eye on the patient's condition and make adjustments to the treatment plan in response to any changes in

symptoms, vital signs, or test findings.

Imparting Solutions for Novel or Seldom Occurring Toxic Exposures

Due to the paucity of knowledge, encounters with novel or uncommon hazardous exposures may provide particular difficulties. Healthcare professionals should proceed cautiously in these circumstances and maintain awareness and readiness:

1. Collaboration with Experts: To obtain knowledge about possible dangerous chemicals and their effects, speak with poison control centers,

toxicologists, or medical professionals with competence in toxicology.

2. Continued Education and Research:
By reading scholarly publications, attending conferences, and taking part in continuing education courses, you may stay current on newly discovered toxins and toxicological discoveries.

3. Risk Assessment: To ascertain the possible harm and intensity of the exposure, carry out a comprehensive risk assessment. Decisions about monitoring, decontamination, and therapy are guided by this assessment.

4. Be Prepared for Unusual Presentations:
Unfamiliar clinical manifestations could result from new poisons. Healthcare professionals should continue to be highly suspicious and take a wide variety of diagnosis into account.

5. Communicate with Colleagues:
Exchange knowledge and firsthand accounts with other medical professionals. Working together might produce ideas and suggestions for handling unusual or unique hazardous exposures.

6. Examine Your Clusters:

Take into consideration the likelihood of a common source or agent if several patients appear with comparable exposures or symptoms. Examine possible clusters to find trends and possible reasons.

Results

Vigilance, knowledge, and teamwork are necessary for managing unknown compounds and new poisons. Healthcare professionals must use a methodical strategy to collect data, administer first care, and modify their plans as circumstances change. New or infrequent toxic exposures can provide challenges that can be met with further knowledge, expert consultation, and a willingness to consider creative solutions. Healthcare professionals can successfully negotiate the complexity of unknown hazardous chemicals and give their patients the best care possible by combining these strategies.